More DEAFINITIONS!

Ken Glickman

Illustrated by Randy Lyhus

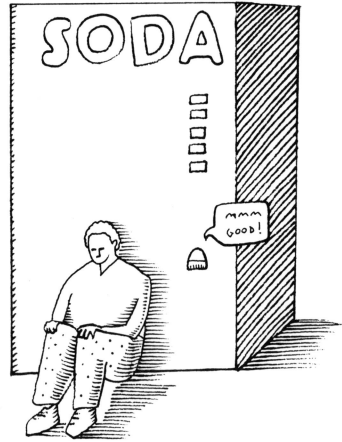

LICKED 'N' KICKED   *(LIKT an KIKT)*
adj. How a previously LICKED 'N' CLICKED DEAFIE really feels after the stubborn vending machine has inexplicably stopped returning his rejected change and his selection never materialized.

More DEAFINITIONS!

For
SIGNLETS*

* Any word pertaining to the world of the deaf that
isn't in the dictionary, but should be.

Published by **DiKen Products**
9201 Long Branch Parkway, Silver Spring, Maryland 20901

More DEAFINITIONS!
First Edition
Text by Ken Glickman
Illustrations by Randy Lyhus

Also by Ken Glickman
DEAFINITIONS For SIGNLETS, the first humor book
  Offers over 265 new words with humorous "deafinitions."
  45 illustrations by Randy Lyhus; 120 pages, paperback.
  Copyright 1986 by Kenneth P. Glickman
  Library of Congress Catalog Card Number 86-72758
  ISBN 0-9617583-0-9
DEAFinitions, the poster
  Contains 50 witty sentences - each using the word, deaf.
  Black on white, 100 lbs. quality gloss paper; Size: 16" by 20"
  Copyright 1986 by DiKen Products

Copyright 1989 by Kenneth P. Glickman
Library of Congress Catalog Card Number 89-50119
ISBN 0-9617583-1-7

Dedicated

to

My two reptilian friends,

IG

Who, on one very warm summer day, left forever through an open window while I was TYPEVERSATING

&

IGU

Whose last favorite meal was a slice of sizzling-hot pizza.

Acknowledgements with Special Thanks

George Balsley

Mamie Bittner

May and David Black

Thomas N. Bland, Jr.

Genie Blatecky

Virgie Bletsch

Bonnie Boswell

Bernard Bragg

Edith David

Mary Davis

Angie Donnell

Diane and Dillip Emmanual

Anita Farb

Robert Giuntoli

Deb Glick

Hilary Goldberg

Bonnie Gracer

Rebecca Hozinsky

Pat Johanson

Russell Kane

Daniel J. Langholtz

Jean Lindquist

Dwight F. Long

Deb Maxwell

Lynn Messing

Marianne K. Moyer

David Officer

Donna Platt

Syria Ponce

Denise M. Reilly

Eric Reisman

Barbara "Babs" Riggs

Rep. Dan Rostenkowski (D-Ill.)

Kenneth G. Samson

Irene Schuchman

Michael W. Schuster, M.D.

Louis Schwarz

Vivienne Simmons

Virginia Spatz

Gail Steever

Joan Stein

Barbara Snyder

Stephen W. Sullivan

Linda Taylor

Jesse Thomas

Jayne Tubergen

Fred S. Weiner

Sharon R. Wilson

And, President George Herbert Walker Bush

Table of Contents

A HEARIE's Foreword

Much has happened in the deaf world since the publication three years ago of *DEAFINITIONS For SIGNLETS*. A deaf actress has been propelled into stardom after winning an Oscar for her role in a movie that tries to show (however imperfectly) the tumultuous meeting of the deaf and hearing worlds. Student demonstrators rocked the campus of Gallaudet University (the only liberal arts college for the deaf in the world). The events leading to the appointment of a deaf president at Gallaudet made national and even international news. Suddenly, deaf people were being interviewed on the nightly news programs.

The exhilaration of the deaf world is further reflected in *More DEAFINITIONS!* Now more than ever we need Ken Glickman to help navigate us between the two worlds. The word "interpreter" appears over and over again in these two *DEAFINITIONS* books. Ken Glickman and *DEAFINITIONS* are the best interpreters that we have to understand what the DEAFIE world is really like and what happens when DEAFIES and HEARIES meet. *DEAFINITIONS* are there to hold a humorous mirror up to ourselves and to show us how hilarious and sometimes painful those encounters can be. Ken Glickman knows just where to hold that mirror because he is an insider who is able to give voice to that world that many of us would otherwise not hear.

Michael W. Schuster, M.D.
Jericho, New York

A DEAFIE'S Foreword

All that is needed to capsulize the developments which have taken place between the publication of Ken Glickman's first book, *DEAFINITIONS For SIGNLETS,* and this one is six words: Marlee Matlin, King Jordan, Gallaudet students. The wondrous world of DEAFIES, as we know it, has changed dramatically.

I must admit, however, that the changes are not necessarily all good. There is so much interest in us DEAFIES that HEARIES are starting to learn Sign Language. A case in point was when I got pulled over (again) by a friendly highway trooper who then proceeded to point out my rather liberal interpretation of the local driving laws. I assumed this was what he was alluding to because I could not understand a word of his speech. In my most winning smile, I wrote on a piece of paper that I was deaf and could he please write everything he just said. I admit, unabashedly, that this was a blatant attempt to manipulate yet another **COP OUT**. Imagine my surprise when he smiled from ear to ear and asked for my driver's license in Sign Language. So you see, it is not all glitter and gold in the Kingdom of the DEAFIES.

Seriously, however, *DEAFINITIONS* is considered by us DEAFIES to be a book that hits home. Where else can you find the definition of **DELAYED REACTION** as described in this book? How many of us DEAFIES have experienced rude stares from other drivers as our cars bob and weave in traffic like a punch-drunk fighter, merely because we were employing the **"LOOK-MAMA-NO-HANDS" TECHNIQUE**? Who else but a DEAFIE can describe in vivid detail the frustration he or she feels while constantly witnessing **COVERT COVERS** on television? I can go on and on, but you get the idea.

There have been numerous books written throughout the years which talk about us DEAFIES. Some books address a broad range of topics and mix empirical evidence along with theories that somehow end up half-baked just the same. Some other books take an historical approach which requires a great deal of research. Finally, there are books in which the author speaks from personal experience. Most of these books are touching, but usually are told from one point of view - the author's. *More DEAFINITIONS!*, however, is one of the few books written about Deaf culture that enables each and every one of us to look at the lighter side of deafness.

Ken is a man of many interests and it is always fascinating to see him hard at work. I have been fortunate enough to observe Ken Glickman in action as he conjured up ideas for this book. You could see the wheels in his head spinning constantly as he came up with yet another situation that we DEAFIES encounter in daily life. His eyes would light up, a strange smile would appear on his face, and he would point a finger in the air and say "I've thought of another word!" His eyes would then frantically roam the room in quest of a pen and paper. This, my friend, is a genius at work.

So remember, have a bag of chips and a bottle of your favorite beverage on hand as you sit back and take a magical tour into the fabulous and wonderful world that we DEAFIES live in.

Enjoy!

Fred S. Weiner
Silver Spring, Maryland

Playing It *Further* by Eye

Ever since *DEAFINITIONS For SIGNLETS* came out a little over two years ago, people have been asking me how I could come up with all those strangely new yet appropriate words. Frankly, I don't have a ready answer, but I think my two good friends, Mike and Steve, have theirs. Steve likes to think that I'm naturally "high," and Mike believes it's because I tend to keep an active and open mind with an alert eye. I daresay only *one* of them is right, or how else can a wordsmith explain it?

My studio is modest. There's this English Pub table that I use as an anvil. Spread about are papers and recipes and small tools. Words first germinate in my mind, and I then snatch a piece of paper and grab a small tool called a felt-tip pen. With the piece atop the anvil and pen in hand, the word is created right there and then. More often than not, the word is coarse and needs more hammering. It's quite amazing how much one can do with a mere twenty six letters of the alphabet let alone all those other special symbols. Words are, fortunately, very malleable. That's why I've had so much fun with them.

Papers make wonderful media with which to carry the fragile words everywhere. Soon after a word is formed on paper, I carry this paper container from the anvil to my electronic fire for further refining. Computers make marvelous machines, and I can't imagine how wordsmiths of bygone times actually managed without them. Once the word reaches its desired form, I take it from the fire to the quenching bucket in an instant. Often known as a laser printer, the bucket freezes the word for the final casting.

Those SIGNLETS cast in boldface caps and embedded in DEAFINITIONS are new and are themselves DEAFINED elsewhere in this book. For all those other SIGNLETS that are capitalized only, they can be found in the first volume, *DEAFINITIONS For SIGNLETS*.

Recipes for inspiration are four dictionaries, three thesauruses, my own personal experiences as a DEAFORMED DEAFIE (and sometimes as a HEAFIE), *A Dictionary of Idioms for the Deaf* by Maxine T. Boatner and John E. Gates (Barron's Educational Series, Inc.), Roy Holcomb's *Silence is Golden Sometimes* (Dawn Sign Press), Rich Hall's *SNIGLETS* and *MORE SNIGLETS* (Collier Books) and tidbits from contributors from every walk of life.

Such is my modest studio. It is where your friendly wordsmith happily churns out new SIGNLETS and DEAFINITIONS day after day and sees them off to that wonderful, majestic world of English, knowing very well that some may not survive for very long, while others might.

Ken Glickman
DEAFinitely Yours Studio
Silver Spring, Maryland
January 15, 1989

More
DEAFINITIONS
and
SIGNLETS

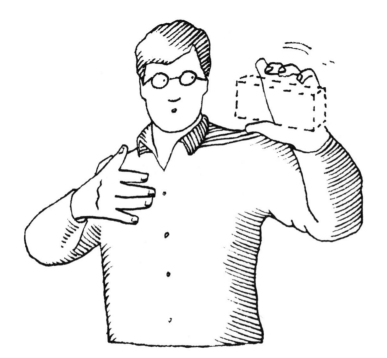

AIRASE
(ay RAYS)

v. To erase **MISFINGERED** words or incorrect signs in the air.

AIRTAP
(ayr tap)

v. To get a DEAFIE's attention by blowing from behind.

ALFRED E. NEUMAN SYNDROME, THE
(al fred ee NEW man SYN drohm)

n. Protruding ears due to oversized hearing aids.

ALL EYES
(AWL YZ)

adj. Very attentive < tell me all about it, I'm ~ >.

ALL THUMBS
(AWL thumz)

adj. Very awkward, especially when first learning the manual alphabet or American Sign Language (ASL).

ALPHANTASY
(al FANT uh see)

n. A bizarre (and often graphic) story told in sign language that uses all the handshapes in the manual alphabet, in order.

AS GOOD AS ONE'S SIGN
(az good az wunz SYN)

adj. phr. Trustworthy.

ASLIANS
(AY ES EL unz)

n. Manualists whose native ~~tongue~~ hand(s) is American Sign Language.

AT A LOSS FOR SIGNS
(at uh LAWS for SYNZ)

adj. phr. How a bewildered HEARIE with a limited Sign vocabulary would feel when accosted by a DEAFIE asking for directions and/or time.

ATMOSTPHERE
(AT MOHST feer)

n. The maximum volume of the sky used by the signer < the ~ of a **BIG HAND** usually takes up the most volume, while the ~ of a DEAFIE baby is often no larger than a watermelon >.

ATTENSTOMP
(uh TEN stomp)

v. To try to get a DEAFIE's attention by stamping one's foot.

ATTENWAVE
(uh TEN wayv)

v. To try to get a DEAFIE's attention by waving. (Note to HEARIES: this is *not* the same as waving good-byes.)

BATTLE OF THE BULGE

(BAT uhl of thuh BUHLJ)

n. A blossoming DEAFIE girl's struggle with BOOBAPPARITION.

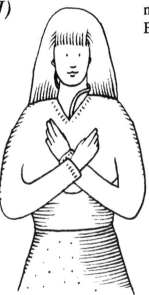

BAWDY LANGUAGE

(BAWD ee LANG gwij)

n. (Same as **BODY LANGUAGE**.)

BEFOREHANDING
(bi FOHR hand ing)

v. (Interpreter jargon) Stretching and wiggling one's hands and fingers prior to interpreting.

BIG HAND
(BIG hand)

n. A boastful, foolish, or **VOSIGNFEROUS** signer.

BING
(bing)

v. (DEAFIE jargon) To tend to; to exhibit an inclination. (See **DEAF WAY**.)

BODY LANGUAGE
(BAWD ee LANG gwij)

n. Nudists' sign language.

BRAIN-FRIED
(BRAYN fryd)

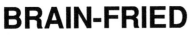

adj. Being electrocuted by a defective hearing aid.

BUSH'S POSTULATE
(bush es PAWS chuh layt)

n. *READ MY LIPS*.
(See **ROSTENKOWSKI'S REFUTATION**.)

BY SIGN OF HAND
(by syn of hand)

adv. phr. How deaf gossip or DEAFAME gets around.

CHAIN REACTION

(chayn ree AK shun)

n. A phenomenon often observed in any gathering of DEAFIES, where everybody eventually turn their attention to a CATCHAJERK.

CHINUPING

(CHIN uhp ing)

v. Keeping one's chin up during a COMFRONTION.

CLEAN ONE'S ATMOSTPHERE

(kleen wunz AT MOHST feer)

v. phr. imperative. To remove elements of **OBSIGNITY** from one's sign language at once.

CLEARIFY

(KLIR uh fy)

v. To free from SIGNFERENCE or obstruction; to make way for COMFRONTION < please ~ your mouth of that ugly cigar >. (Compare with FLOWER-REARRANGE.)

COLD HANDS

(kohld handz)

n. That temporary, paralyzing loss of self-confidence prior to interpreting.

COLD TURKEY

(kohld TER kee)

n. A HEARIE who, after his very first sign language lesson, jumps right into a DEAFIE social gathering and awkwardly signs to everyone "HI."

CONSCIOUSNESS RAZING

(KON chuh snuhs RAYZ ing)

n. That remarkable week-long phenomenon in March 1988, where the entire world woke up to the clamor at Gallaudet University.

COP OUT

(KOP OUT)

v. To refrain from issuing speeding tickets to DEAFIE drivers and D.D.D.'s.

COP'S DILEMMA

(kops duh LEM uh)

v. To arrest or not to arrest a group of marching DEAFIES on a street.

COVERT COVERS
(KOH vert KUV erz)

n. Those most annoying TV decoder's captions that either conceal a network's own captions or discreetly shield a pretty actress's cleavage from view.

CRAB-WALKING
(krab wawk ing)

v. Walking sideways and COMFRONTING at the same time.

CRANIUM CRUSHER
(KRAY nee uhm KRUHSH er)

n. A pair of cumbersome, heavy, old-fashioned headphones.

CRANIUM INDENTUS
(KRAY nee um in DENT us)

n. A pathological condition found among DEAFIE kids, whose heads are caved in from the top due to prolonged use of a **CRANIUM CRUSHER**.

CROONING MOONBEAMS
(kroon ing MOON beemz)

n. Those soft beams of light seeping into a completely dark bedroom - vital for a cozy COMFRONTION.

DEAF ARM
(DEF arm)

n. That seemingly dead limb of a DEAFIE, who doesn't respond to ATTENTAPPING. (Usually marked by a few ugly TAPCRATERS.)

DEAF CULTURE
(DEF KUL chur)

n. A wonderful way of life that is unheard of. (Note to all Biologists: This term does *not* mean DEAFIES DEAFORMED *in vitro*.)

DEAF LEADING THE DEAF

(DEF leed ing thuh DEF)

n. phr. An oralist **MISUNDERSHANDING** for another.

DEAF WAY, THE

(DEF way)

n. What DEAFIES **BING**.

DEAFECTIVE

(def FEK tive)

adj. What manualists, oralists, and **SIMULISTS** all call each other.

DEAFENSE

(de FENS)

n. That menacing line of Gallaudet University football players.

DEAFGATE
(DEF gayt)

n. Coverup of discrimination of DEAFIES by the DEAF-IMPAIRED.

DEAFIE BEETHOVEN
(DEF ee BAY toh vun)

n. An endearing term usually reserved for one's DEAFIE kid < someday he'll become ~, he's so good at it. >.

DEAFIE WIDOW (-ER)
(DEF ee WID oh, WID uh wer)

n. A HEARIE whose spouse spends much time playing in the deaf world.

DEAFILE
(def FYL)

v. Exactly what **OUTCLAWS** do to ASL.

DEAFING AID
(DEF ing ayd)

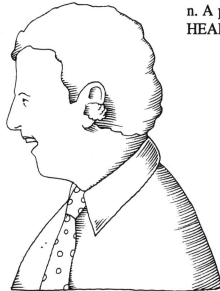

n. A pair of cotton wads sticking out of a HEARIE's ears.

DEAFISTIC
(DEF is TIK)

adj. That admirable quality of acting and looking just like a DEAFIE. (Applies to DEARIES only.)

DEAFOLOGIST
(DEF uh LOH just)

n. One who studies all these little quirks of DEAFIES and their interactions with HEARIES, HEAFIES, and DEARIES.

DEAFORMITY
(de FORM i tee)

n. Any grotesquely shaped part of a DEAFIE's anatomy. (See the **DELTA** group below.)

DECODING THE DECODER
(DEE coh ding thuh DEE coh der)

v. phr. Trying frantically to figure out how to hookup the closed-captioned decoder with the VCR and TV.

DEEPEENOW
(DEE PEE NOW)

n. A DEAFIE's battle cry for a Deaf President.

DELAYED REACTION
(dee layd REE ak shun)

n. A TV situation with closed-captioned programs, where DEAFIES tend to laugh after HEARIES are finished.

DELTA ARM (△A)
(DEL tuh arm)

n. (Physiology) That little noticeable difference in arm lengths of a DEAFIE, where one is longer due to excessive **ATTENWAVING**.

DELTA DEAFIE (ΔD)
(DEL tuh DEF ee)

n. That little noticeable difference in the overall appearance of DEAFIES and DEARIES that sets them apart.

DELTA EAR (ΔE)
(DEL tuh EER)

n. That little noticeable difference in the NO-MOLD ZONES in the ears of a DEAFIE, where one is larger due to excessive wearing of the earmold.

DELTA FOOT (ΔF)
(DEL tuh foot)

n. That little noticeable difference in the breadth of feet of a DEAFIE, where one is wider due to excessive ATTENSTOMPING on the floor.

DELTA HAND (ΔH)
(DEL tuh hand)

n. That little noticeable difference in the overall size of the hands of a DEAFIE, where one is larger due to being right-handed or left-handed.

DESIGNATE
(DEZ ig nayt)

v. To single out DEAFIE pre-schoolers for oral deaf schools.

DESIGNER
(di ZY ner)

n. One who attempts to convert manualists to oralists. (Compare with **MUTELATOR**.)

DISARMING
(dis ARM ing)

v. What a **DESIGNER** does to manualists.

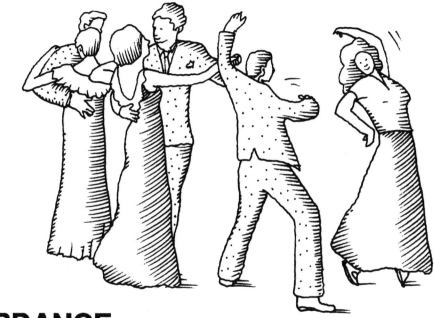

DISCORDANCE

(dis kor DANS)

n. A strange ritual often observed at discos, where DEAFIES dance slowly to some fast music (and vice versa).

33

DISVOCALIZE
(dis VOH kuh lyz)

v. To mouth words (in conjunction with one's signing).

DOUBLE-QUIET
(DUB bul KWY et)

adj. How a DEAFIE actually feels in a silent, dark place.

DRUM-HIKE
(DRUM hyk)

v. (Football jargon) To commence a football play on the field in an instant response to the banging of the **PSEUDO-VOICEBOX**.

DRY SENSE OF HAND
(dry sens of HAND)

n. Subtle humor in sign language.

D.S.T.
(DEE ES TEE)

n. Deaf Standard Time, a temporal system used by DEAFIES, where they tend to arrive one hour to two hours after a party has started.

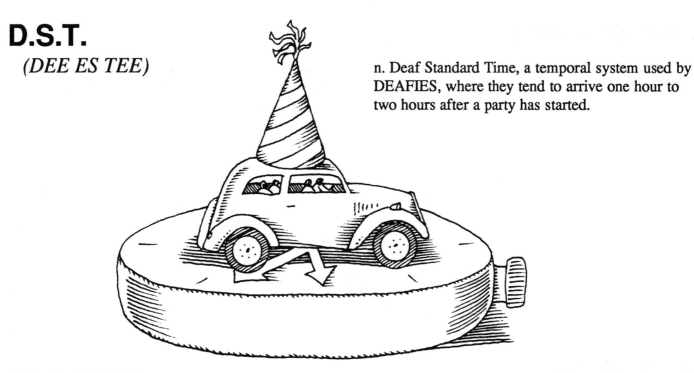

EAR-MISS
(EER mis)

n. The reason why interpreters sign "Four there..." when the speaker actually said "For their...."

EAR-OPENER

(EER op uh ner)

n. (Applicable to HEARIES only) Something very surprising or startling. (Note: "Eye-opener" is applicable to DEAFIES only.)

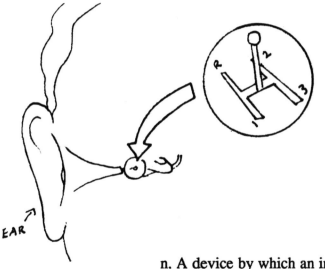

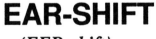

EAR-SHIFT

(EER shift)

n. A device by which an interpreter's hearing is automatically engaged and disengaged while interpreting between a HEARIE and a manualist.

EAR-STRAIN
(EER strayn)

n. The reason why interpreters charge DEAFIES with high **HEARNINGS**.

EARLING
(EER ling)

n. A HEARIE animal one year old.

EARRESISTABLE
(IR i ZIS tuh buhl)

adj. The reason why HEARIES are often drawn to the sound of DEAFIES' **OBVOICE** and also why everyone EARSNIFFS these days.

EARRIGATING
(IR uh gayt ing)

v. Flooding one's hearing aid while swimming (often after experiencing AQUASHOCK).

EARRITATED
(IR i tay ted)

adj. How one feels after he has been EARSNIFFED by somebody who happens to find his **ALFRED E. NEUMAN SYNDROME EARRESISTABLE.**

EARTHQUACK
(UHRTH KWAK)

n. A DEAFIE found banging and kicking on his sleeping DEAFIE friend's door in an apartment building (instead of a natural disaster as first thought by all the other tenants).

EASY-OF-DEAF
(EE zee of def)

adj. hard-of-hearing or SOFT-OF-DEAF.

EE-ATTACK

(EE uh TAK)

n. A chronic or recurrent outburst of high-pitched whistling emitted from a DEAFIE's hearing aid.

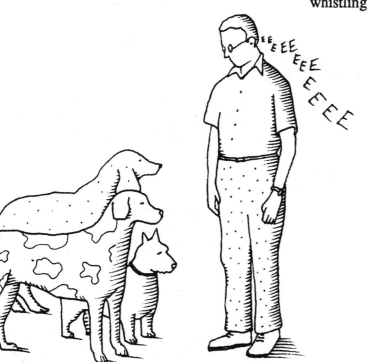

EEK-ATTACK
(EEK uh TAK)

n. A HEARIE stranger's sudden shock in response to a DEAFIE's **EE-ATTACK**.

ELECTRO-VAPORIZATION
(i LEK troh vay puhr uh ZAY shun)

n. A gradual, nocturnal process that commences when DEAFIES forget to turn off the overhead light inside the car after AUTOBABBLING.

EXCUSE PRINCIPLE, THE
(ik SKYEWS PRIN suh puhl)

n. What devious DEAFIES often employ when caught in an QUEUEVASION, saying "I didn't know, I didn't hear, I can't hear, I am deaf,...."

EYEDDICT
(Y dikt)

n. A person with a pathological condition prevalent among DEAFIES ENRAPTIONED by TV-watching.

EYED
(yd)

v. (Past tense) Heard via one's eyes.

EYETH
(yth)

n. What this planet of ours would be called had there been far more DEAFIES than HEARIES.

FACEDOWNING
(FAYS down ing)

v. Talking to the floor instead of **CHINUPING** to a DEAFIE.

FACELIFTING
(FAYS lif ting)

v. Telling a HEARIE **FACEDOWNER** to please **CHINUP** while COMFRONTING.

FACELITATE
(fay SIL uh tayt)

v. To make it easier for a nice COMFRONTION with DEAFIES.

FACEVALUE
(FAYS val ew)

n. Degree of expressiveness and legibility of the speaker's countenance < one is said to have a good ~ if he is easy to lipread or to be understood by DEAFIES >.

FAXPRESSION
(FAKS pres shun)

n. (Telecommunications jargon) All those typed expressions, such as "SMILE", "SMACK", "HA HA", "GOSH", and "GEE".

FINGERBITE
(FING ur byt)

n. A winter-time affliction found chiefly among manual DEAFIES who agonize every time they try to spell out in the cold air.

FINGERPAINTING
(FING ur PAYN ting)

n. A DEAFIE kid's version of **HANDSCAPE**.

FINGER-SLICKIN' GOOD
(FING ur SLIK in good)

adj. Fluent in fingerspelling.

FINGERTIP-OFF
(FING ur TIP of)

n. That tell-tale hand movement that reveals one is not simply gesturing, but signing.

FLASHFLUSH
(FLASH FLUSH)

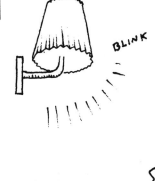

v. To tell a **PREOCCUPIED** DEAFIE in a bathroom to please hurry up whatever he/she is doing by repeatedly flashing the light inside from outside.

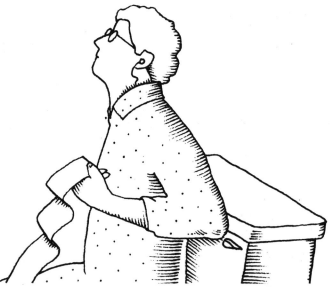

FLYATTENTAP
(fly uh TEN tap)

v. To attract attention of a DEAFIE by throwing something at him.

FORCING ONE'S HAND
(fors ing wunz HAND)

v. phr. Trying to convert a reluctant oralist to a manualist.

FOUR EARS
(FOR eerz)

n. A derogatory term sometimes used to describe a person with two hearing aids.

FREUDIAN SIGN
(FROY dee uhn SYN)

n. A misplaced, and possibly offensive, sign.

FRONT-SEAT DRIVER
(fruhnt seet DRY ver)

n. A passenger steering the car and signing with his free right hand so that the DEAFIE driver with his foot still on the gas pedal can watch him instead of the road.

GA-GA-GA
(GEE AY GEE AY GEE AY)

v. (Telecommunications jargon) What a **TYPEVERSATOR** says to an **UNGACIOUS TYPEVERSATOR** at the other end of the line.

GENE MUTEATION THEORY
(JEEN MEWT ay shuhn THEE uh ree)

n. (Biology) A theory that attempts to explain why some DEAFIE babies grow up to be oralists and others to be manualists.

GROUND-ZERO
(grownd ZEER oh)

n. That exact spot where an **ATTENSTOMPING** DEAFIE's foot meets the floor.

GUESSTURES
(GES chuhrz)

n. International sign language.

H-BOMB
(AYCH BOM)

n. A television set with loudness volume left preset to "Maximum" by a DEAFIE and later detonated by an unwitting HEARIE.

HAIDE 'N' EEK
(hyd en EEK)

n. A perplexing game that a DEAFIE child plays with parents, where the kid's hearing aid is left on and buried in a pile of clothes or even in a sandbox and parents go crazy trying to find the source of the annoying whistling sound.

HAND-EYE COORDINATION
(HAND y koh or duh NAY shun)

n. (Communication jargon) What transpires between a manualist and a HEARIE.

HANDFUL
(HAND ful)

adj. How a waitress/waiter feels when serving a large gathering of signing, dining DEAFIES.

HANDICAP
(HAN dee kap)

n. Disability of HEARIES that somehow prevents them from signing gracefully.

HANDICAPPED
(HAN dee kapt)

adj. How a manualist with two broken wrists really feels.

HAND IN HAND
(HAND in HAND)

exp. How two DEAFIE lovers WHISPIGN sweet nothings to each other in total darkness.

HANDS ARE SMALLER THAN ONE'S STOMACH

(HANDZ ayr SMAWL ler than wunz STUHM uhk)

exp. What DEAFIE kids always exclaim when issued a **MOTHER'S ADMONITION.**

HANDSCAPE

(HAND skayp)

n. An imaginative and often poetic scenery created solely by signing in ASL.

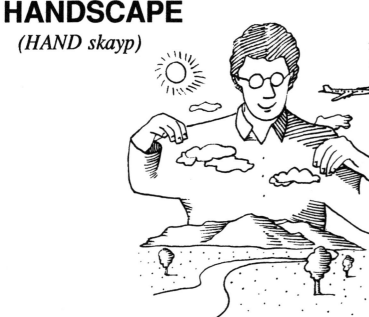

HANDS-DOWN
(HANDZ down)

adj. Very easy. (Note: This applies *only* to those oralists with excellent lipreading skills.)

HANDSLIDE
(HAND slyd)

n. (Sign language class jargon) An overpowering movement of a mass of new, fresh signs.

HANDSOME
(HAN suhm)

adj. 1. Very beautiful in signing.
-LY adv. 2. Too much.

HANDWRITING
(HAND ry ting)

v. Signing in the air.

HANDY
(HAN dee)

adj. Adept in signing.

HAPPY NEW EAR!
(HAP pee new EER)

exp. A greeting usually reserved for a DEAFIE who just became a PHONYPHONIC.

HARASS-EMBARRASS
(huh RAS im BAR uhs)

v. To unintentionally tap on a stranger's shoulder (or bosom) in a public place, thinking he/she was your deaf shopping companion.

HAWAIIANED
(huh WAW yuhnd)

adj. A term that best describes an interpreter who ought to know better than to wear a colorful, splashy T-shirt.

HEAR AND KNOW
(HEER and NOH)

v. phr. To catch that tell-tale **OBVOICE** of a DEAFIE on that very spot at that very instant.

HEARACHE
(HEER ayk)

n. Sorrow brought about by wishing one were hearing.

HEARBROKEN
(HEER broh kun)

adj. Overcome by **HEARACHE**.

HEARCULEAN
(HEER kyuh lee uhm)

adj. Of extraordinary endurance and perseverance to succeed in the hearing world.

HEAREDITY
(hee RED uht ee)

n. (Same as **INHEARITANCE.**)

HEARESY
(HEER uh see)

n. An unthinkable thought of a **HEARETIC.**

HEARETIC
(HEER uh tik)

n. A dissenter in the world of the deaf.

HEARING-AIDE
(HEER ing ayd)

n. A DEAFIE helping a HEARIE understand all those little quirks of sign language.

HEARING-IMPAIRED
(HEER ing im PAYRD)

adj. A term that aptly describes HEARIES who could, but don't, hear DEAFIES.

HEARING LOSS
(HEER ing los)

n. Sudden withdrawal of a **HEARMIT** from a social gathering of one too many DEAFIES.

HEARLY BIRD
(HEER lee BIRD)

n. A HEARIE that "catches the word" ahead of DEAFIES.

HEARMARK
(HEER mark)

v. To **"DESIGNATE"** some young DEAFIES for MINORSTREAMING in hearing public schools.

HEARMIT
(HEER muht)

n. A HEARIE who retreats from the deaf world.

HEAR-MUFFS
(HEER mufs)

n. (Same as **DEAFING AID**.)

HEARNEST
(HEER nist)

a. A term that best describes a HEAFIE.

HEARNINGS

(HEER ningz)

n. That inexorably high fee interpreters charge DEAFIES for their understanding of HEARIES by listening. (Compare with **INVOICE**.)

HEARO

(HEE roh)

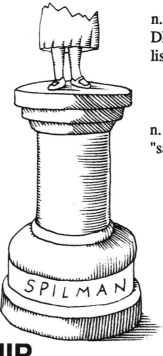

n. A HEARIE who mistakenly thinks he is out to "save" DEAFIES.

HEARO WORSHIP

(HEE roh wur shup)

(There is no such thing in the world of the deaf.)

HEARPLUGS

(HEER pluhgz)

n. (Same as **DEAFING AID**.)

HEARSPLITTING

(HEER split ing)

adj. What a **HEARMIT** experiences with a **HEARING LOSS**.

HEAR TODAY, GONE TOMORROW

(HEER too DAY GAWN too MAH roh)

n. exp. 1. Deafness, as a result of the aging process. 2. What inevitably happens to all of us anyway.

HESISTATION

(hez uh STAY shun)

adj. That guilty feeling a **HEARIE** passenger experiences in a **DEAFIE**'s car while debating with himself whether to use the car radio.

HIPCRATER
(HIP kray ter)

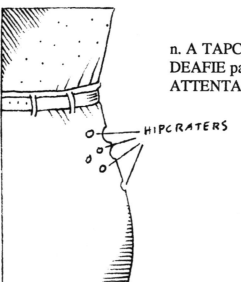

HIPCRATERS

n. A TAPCRATER found on the waistline of a DEAFIE parent caused by an UNCONTACTFUL, ATTENTAPPING child.

HUNCH BACK OF NOTED FAME
(HUHNCH BAK of NOHT uhd FAYM)

n. A crooked-back **TYPEVERSATOR** with an uncanny intuitive ability to foretell what you were about to type on a TDD.

HYENAING

(hy EE nuh ing)

v. Opening and closing one's hand(s) repetitively - alternating between the "H" and "A" handshapes - while laughing.

ILLEGAL ALIENS

(i LEE guhl AYL yuhnz)

n. Those wild animals living in the attic and basement unbeknownst to the DEAFIE homeowner.

IN ONE EYE AND OUT THE OTHER

(in wun Y and owt thuh UHTH er)

adv. phr. Not paying attention.

INDIGESIGNATION
(in dee JES syn a chun)

n. A pathological condition often afflicting DEAFIES causing heartburn when trying to assimilate new sign language variations imparted to them by HEARIES.

INFLATED TOUCH-TONE
(in FLAYT ed TUCH tohn)

n. That "loudly" vibrating balloon found in the hands of DEAFIE spectators during a musical performance.

INHEARITANCE
(in HEER uht uhns)

n. A HEARIE child of a DEAFIE parent.

INHEARITANCE TAX
(in HEER uht uhns TAKS)

n. A certain percentage of the value of family jewels that is levied on HEARIES for the privilege of being able to hear.

INSIGNT
(IN synt)

n. What usually distinguishes manualists from HEARIES and oral DEAFIES in their intuitive UNDERSHANDING of ASL and all its little quirks.

INVISIBLE EARICAP
(in VIZ uh bul EER ee kap)

n. Hearing.

INVISIBLE HANDICAP
(in VIZ uh bul HAN dee kap)

n. Deafness.

INVOICE
(IN voys)

n. That inexorably high fee interpreters charge HEARIES for their **UNDERSHANDING** of manualists in voice. (Compare with **HEARNINGS**.)

IT LOOKS GOOD
(it luks good)

exp. It sounds good.

JAWBREAKER

(JAW bray ker)

n. A lousy speech therapist.

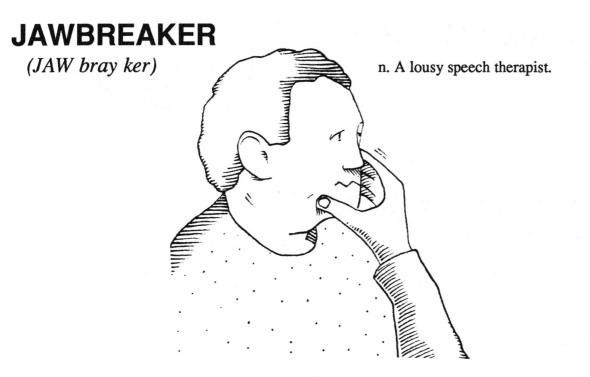

JOHN-HANCOCKIZE

(JAWN HAN kawk yz)

v. To sign in a grandiose fashion.

JOWLY SYNDROME, THE

(JAW lee SYN droym)

n. A pathological condition of having saggy flesh in the area of the lower jaw due to prolonged speech training with a **JAWBREAKER**.

KEEP ONE'S HANDS SHUT

(KEEP wunz handz SHUT)

v. phr. imperative. To shut up.

KICK NICK

(KIK NIK)

n. One of those unsightly marks on the bottom part of a DEAFIE's front door - often caused by **EARTHQUACKS**.

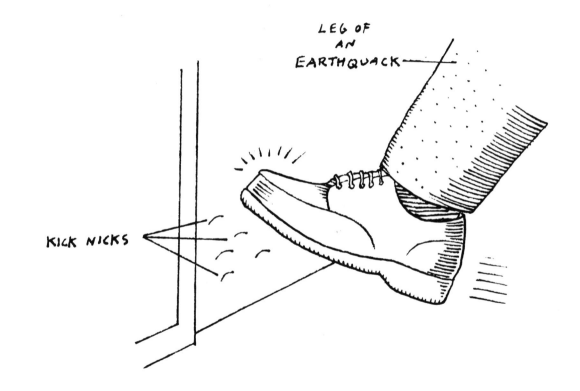

KIDTAP
(KID tap)

v. To snatch a hearing kid's attention in order to get attention of a DEAFIE child.

KING'S ENGLISH
(KINGZ ING glish)

n. The proper speech and usage of English and what got our beloved King his present job at Gallaudet University.

KING'S RANSOM
(kingz RAN sum)

n. The Office of Presidency at Gallaudet University.

LENDING ONE'S HAND
(lend ing wunz HAND)

v. phr. The reason why interpreters get paid **HANDSOMELY**.

LICENSE-PLATING
(LYS uhns PLAYT ing)

v. Typing on TDD in an abbreviated or condensed manner, such as "U OK?", "THANX", "U 2", and "ALL 4 NOW."

LICKED 'N' KICKED
(LIKT an KIKT)

adj. How a previously LICKED 'N' CLICKED DEAFIE really feels after the stubborn vending machine has inexplicably stopped returning his rejected change and his selection never materialized.

LIGHT-FINGERED
(LYT FING gerd)

adj. What you call one who just **TOOK SIGNS RIGHT OUT OF YOUR HANDS**.

LOCAL VOCAL FOCAL POINT

(LOH kuhl VOH kuhl FOH kuhl POYNT)   n. That elusive spot in a group, where a DEAFIE or HEARIE can see and understand all others.

LONGHAND

(LONG hand)   n. Normal signing with everything signed and spelled out.

LOOK-ALIKES

(luk uh LYKS)   n. PHIPHTHEENS, such as "bee" and "me," and "six" and "sex".

"LOOK-MAMA-NO-HANDS" TECHNIQUE, THE

(luk MA ma noh handz tek NEEK)   n. A method sometimes employed by deaf car drivers, in which they sign to their passengers with their two free hands while their knees handle the steering wheel.

LOUD HAND
(LOWD hand)

n. (Same as **BIG HAND**.)

LOWJACK
(LOH jak)

v. To commandeer Gallaudet University buses, hotwire and park them by the gates, and slash the tires as was done during the "Deaf President Now" Protest. (Note to all oral DEAFIES: Compare with "Hijack," which is, incidentally, *not* a salutatory greeting.)

MANUAL FAILURE
(MAN yew al FAYL yuhr)

n. A HEARIE who can do anything but sign.

MANUAL TEST

(MAN yew al test)

n. A substitute exam **UNDESIGNED** especially for **ASLIANS** who loathe oral tests.

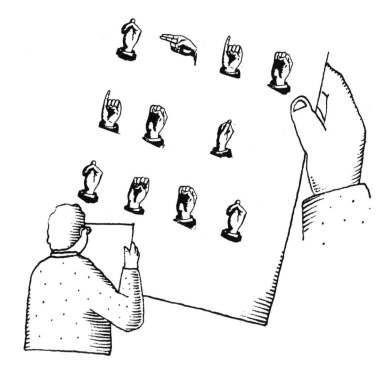

MANUALIST'S AXIOM

(MAN yew al ests AKS see uhm)

n. Signs speak louder than words. (Compare with **ORALIST'S AXIOM** and **SIMULIST'S AXIOM.**)

MICROWAVE

(MIK roh wayv)

v. To wave with the pinky finger.

MINCING ONE'S SIGNS

(MINS ing wunz synz)

n. Saying very little with hands.

MISFINGERED

(mis FING erd)

adj. Not spelled correctly in the air by hand.

MISTALKE

(mi STAWK)

v. To misinterpret or **MISUNDERSHAND** < Don't ~ me, I mean exactly what I signed >.

MISUNDERSHAND

(mis un der SHAND)

v. 1. To fail to comprehend one's signing. 2. To interpret incorrectly one's signing.

MISUNDERSHANDING
(mis un der SHAND ing)

n. Misinterpretation by sign language interpreters.

MOMMY SPILMAN
(MOM mee SPIL man)

n. 1. Endearing nickname for Ms. Jane B. Spilman (*formerly* the Chairwoman of the Gallaudet University Board of Trustees). 2. Any HEARIE held responsible for **PATERNALISPUS**.

MOTHER'S ADMONITION
(MUHTH erz ad MON i shun)

n. "Don't talk with your hands full!"

MOTOR-HAND

(MOH tur hand)

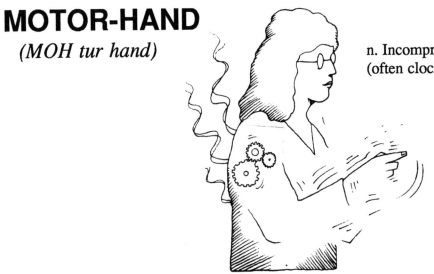

n. Incomprehensible hand movements in ASL (often clocked at 75 MPH).

MURPHY'S LAW OF SIGNBLASTING

(MUR feez law of SYN blast ing)

n. An annoying phenomenon observed often in restaurants, where each DEAFIE diner establishes his own SIGNBLAST RADIUS only to have a DEAFIE fellow sitting next to him knock over his favorite drink.

MUSICKLY
(mew ZIK lee)

adj. How a DEAFIE with an IDIOT'S NOD really feels when told an unfamiliar name of a very popular song or singer.

MUTELATOR
(MYEWT uhl ayt er)

n. One who tries to convert oralists to manualists. (Compare with **DESIGNER**.)

MY SIGNIFICANT OTHER
(my sig NIF i kuhnt UHTH er)

n. One's interpreter.

NEANDERTHALIZE
(nee AN der thah LYZ)

v. To contort one's own face in the mistaken belief that a COMFRONTING DEAFIE would understand better.

NETTED GUY

(net ted gy)

n. That poor DEAFIE sitting between two signing companions trying futilely to follow the conversation. Note: prolonged exposure to this unhealthy situation often leads to TENNIS NECK.

NOTNOWNOTNOW

(NOT noh NOT noh)

n. The feeling one gets when he has his hands full (such as with grocery bags) and sees his DEAFIE friend approaching him.

OBSIGNITY
(ob SYN i tee)

n. Gross, vulgar ASL signs.

OBVOICE
(AWB voys)

n. That peculiar vocal quality of DEAFIES that makes it obvious they are deaf.

OFOR?
(of or, uh for)

n. What one keeps asking while deciding whether an organization's name ends with "of the Deaf" or "for the Deaf."

OLD 'N' COLD
(ohld en kohld)

adj. How the food on a DEAFIE's plate tastes after two hours of signing incessantly at the dinner table.

ON THE HOOK

(ahn thuh HOOK)

adj. phr. How one really feels when he finally learns the DEAFIE's phone he has been trying to ring for hours was off the hook.

ONE'S EYES ARE BURNING

(wunz YZ ayr buhrn ing)

exp. When a DEAFIE feels somebody is signing about him.

ONE'S SIGNS FELL ON HEARING EYES

(wunz SYNZ FEL on HEER ing YZ)

exp. What DEAFIES always say of **SUPERSONIC** HEARIES.

OPTICAL OPTIMALITY

(AWP ti kuhl awp tuh MAL uht ee)

n. What all DEAFIES strive for in **SEESONING**.

ORAL FIXATION
(OHR uhl fik SAY shun)

n. (Psychological/pathological term) A deep-seated condition found only among oral DEAFIES that manifests itself after a prolonged session with a **JAWBREAKER.**

ORALIST'S AXIOM
(OHR uhl ists AKS ee uhm)

n. Word is mightier than sign. (Compare with **MANUALIST'S AXIOM** and **SIMULIST'S AXIOM.**)

OUT OF EYESHOT
(OWT of Y shot)

adj. Being in a DEAFIE's DARF SIDE.

OUT OF SIGHT, OUT OF MIND
(OWT of syt OWT of mynd)

adj. phr. Exactly how a DEAFIE feels during a lecture where there is no interpreter or there is an EYESOGRE sitting in front.

OUTCLAWS
(OWT klawz)

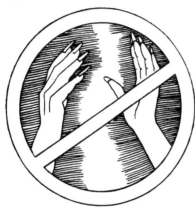

n. 1. Interpreters with colorful and distracting fingernails, who do not abide by their sacred Code of Ethics. 2. Manualists with **UNSIGNTLY** long fingernails.

OUTSPIGNEN
(owt SPYN uhn)

adj. "Outspoken" in signs.

OVERHEAD PROJECTION
(oh ver HED pruh JEK shun)

n. formal. What a DEAFIE student always undergoes in a HEARIE classroom when his interpreter does not show up and the constant verbal stream of the professor's lecture flies right over the DEAFIE's head.

PARABLE PARADOX
(PAR uh buhl PAR uh doks)

n. A seemingly self-contradictory situation where **MANUALIST'S AXIOM, ORALIST'S AXIOM,** and **SIMULIST'S AXIOM** all appear to be true.

PATERNALISPUS
(pa TUR na lis pus)

n. That emotional ooze of disgust that dwells up from inside, such as when DEAFIES in the middle of protesting are told by **MOMMY SPILMAN** to go home and have a good night's sleep.

PEER PRESSURE
(peer PRESH er)

n. The reason why a lone DEAFIE feels compelled to keep focusing on the boring interpreter in a HEARIE classroom. (Compare with **STARE FORCE**.)

PENNED
(pend)

v. (Past tense) Corralled by a DEAFIE asking for a pen or pencil.

PERIPHERAL THRESHOLD
(puh RIF uh ruhl THRESH oyld)

n. That cutoff angle from the front of a DEAFIE, beyond which he cannot be **WAVEATTENED**.

PIDGIN-HOLE
(PID gin hoyl)

v. To classify a signer as a DEAFIE, HEARIE, DEARIE or HEAFIE.

PIERCED EAR

(PIRSD EER)

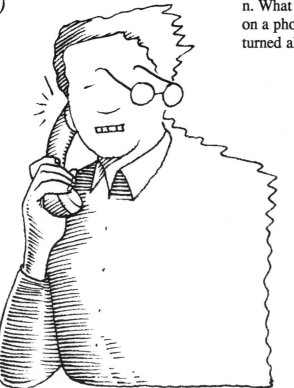

n. What an unwitting HEARIE gets from listening on a phone whose amplifier has been previously turned all the way up by an **EASY-OF-DEAF** user.

PIGGY-BACK RIDER

(PIG ee bak RID er)

n. A HEARIE sitting in a front-row section reserved for DEAFIES at a theater.

POUND BARRIER

(POUND BAR ee er)

n. That invisible wall of DEAFIE resistance to HEARIES' encroachment.

POUND BOOM

(POUND boom)

n. An earth-shaking shock wave created by a fat **ATTENSTOMPER.**

POUND WAVES

(POUND wayvz)

n. Those invisible waves of vibrations radiating outward from **GROUND ZERO** underneath the foot of an **ATTENSTOMPER**, traveling through the floor at the **SPEED OF POUND**.

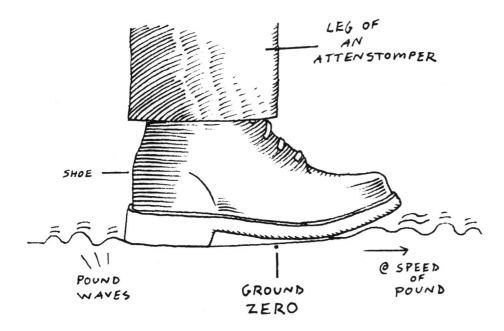

LEG OF
AN
ATTENSTOMPER

SHOE

POUND
WAVES

GROUND
ZERO

@ SPEED
OF
POUND

POUNDING BOARD

(POUND ing bord)

n. A DEAFIE whom HEARIES sometimes pound for his INSIGNT. (Compare with **SOUNDING BOARD**.)

POUNDING HEADACHE

(POUND ing hed ak)

n. A discomfort brought about by excessive **ATTENSTOMPING** by others.

POUNDPROOF

(POUND proof)

adj. Impervious to **POUND WAVES**; having no or very low **SENSITIVITY GRADIENT** < ground is ~, you have to **ATTENWAVE** >.

PREOCCUPIED
(pree OK yuh pyd)

adj. How a DEAFIE really feels while minding her/his business in a restroom whose door has neither a lock nor a sign that says "Occupied."

PROFOUNDLY HEARING
(pruh FOWND lee HEER ing)

adj. phr. 1. (Medical jargon) A term that fits those HEARIES, who resort to incoherent babbling once they lose themselves in the noisy world of the deaf. 2. (Political jargon) A term that best describes Ms. Jane Spilman.

PSEUDO-VOICEBOX
(SOO doh voys boks)

n. That bulky drum on a football-field sideline used mainly for **DRUM-HIKING**.

PUNCHSIGN
(PUHNCH syn)

n. A punchline in sign language.

PUNCHUATION
(PUHN CHUH way shun)

n. What a DEAFIE feels like doing after six grueling hours of English lessons - knock out his teacher.

PUTTING ONE'S FOOT IN ONE'S HANDS
(PUT ting wunz foot in wunz handz)

v. phr. Signing carelessly or signing something you wished you didn't.

PUTTING ONE'S HAND IN ONE'S MOUTH

(PUT ting wunz hand in wunz MOWTH) v. phr. Talking with DEAFACEMENT.

PUTTING SIGNS INTO ONE'S HANDS

(PUT ting SYNZ in too wunz handz) v. phr. What a not-so-honest signer sometimes does on a DEAFIE's DARF SIDE.

QUODA

(KWOH duh) n. A **TOKENIZED** DEAFIE worker.

READER'S INDIGESTION

(REED erz in dy JES chun) n. What a DEAFIE student often experiences in a CLASSIC CLASSROOM CLASHING, where he could not digest all the boring information from his teacher, interpreter, and notetaker - let alone an opened copy of his favorite *Reader's Digest*.

RECEDING CHAIRLINE
(ree SEED ing CHAR lyn)

n. The circular formation of chairs being pushed back from a classroom's center in deaf schools.

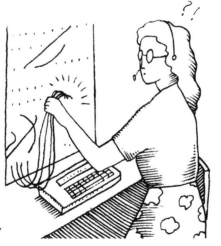

RELAY DELAY
(ree LAY dee LAY)

n. That annoying "bottleneck" at deaf relay message services, where one too many DEAFIES want to make a phone call at the same time.

RELIEF BITCHER
(ri LEEF BICH er)

n. (Deaf institution jargon, archaic) A dormitory housemother who checks you off each time you emerge from a bathroom stall and who has the nerve to ask you whether it's "#1" or "#2."

ROAD SIGNS
(ROHD SYNZ)

n. Exaggerated signs used by D.D.D.'s and SUPERCHATTERS.

ROARTAP
(ROHR tap)

v. To get a SOFT-OF-DEAF DEAFIE's attention by shouting.

ROSTENKOWSKI'S REFUTATION
(ras ten KOW skeez ref yuh TAY shun)

n. *I CAN'T READ LIPS.*
(See **BUSH'S POSTULATE**.)

RUNNING THE GAUNTLET

(RUHN ning thuh GAWNT lit)

v. phr. Trying to COMMUNAVIGATE through a crowded place full of teeming manualists and emerge from this perilous ARMED ZONE unscathed.

SAWED-OFF

(SAWD awf)

adj. How a DEAFIE feels in a BERMUDEAF TRIANGLE.

SECRET SERVICE

(SEE krit SER vis)

n. That corps of interpreters with their very strict Code of Ethics.

SEEPAGE

(SEE pij)

n. An annoying situation that often takes place at airports, where one somehow loses one's DEAFIE companion and can not page him.

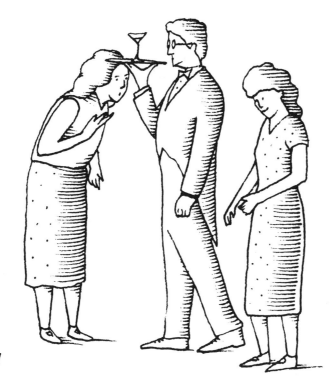

SEESAW
(SEE saw)

n. An on-again, off-again communication struggle between two DEAFIES in a crowded place with lots of SIGNFERENCE.

SEESCAPE

(SEE skayp)

n. That gorgeous, artistic expanse of a **SIGNIFICANT FIGURE**'s **ATMOSTPHERE**.

SEESICKNESS

(SEE sik nuhs)

n. What a **TOKENIZED** DEAFIE often experiences in the dry and boring world of the hearing.

SEESONING

(SEE zon ing)

n. Anything that helps brighten up a room, such as candles, a fireplace, lights, and SOLARMS.

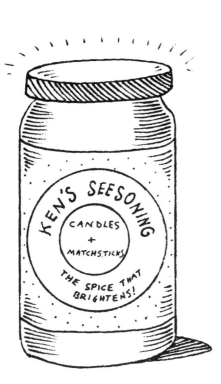

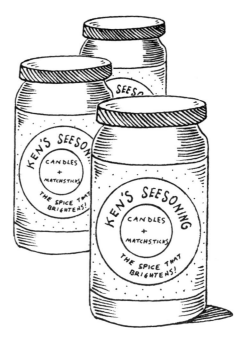

SEE-THRU
(SEE threw)

adj. Possessing an excellent **FACEVALUE**, so good that an oral DEAFIE can lipread right through.

SEEWORTHY
(SEE wer thee)

adj. Fit or safe for lipreading.

SELF-DEAFENSE
(SELF de FENS)

n. The act of retreating after being **SAWED-OFF** in a BERMUDEAF TRIANGLE.

SENSITIVITY GRADIENT
(sen suh TIV uht ee GRAYD ee uhnt)

n. The quality of transmitting vibrations through a medium < hardwood floors have a higher ~ than carpeted floors >.

SENSITIVITY THRESHOLD
(sen suh TIV uht ee THRESH old)

n. The cutoff level of a DEAFIE's ability to sense floor vibration, below which he cannot be **STOMPATTENED.**

SENTENCED
(SEN tensd)

adj. How an interpreter feels after "voicing" a DEAFIE's long-winded sentence in ASL, thinking how great a job he has done until the DEAFIE ends it with a "not."

SHORT-CHANGER
(SHORT CHAYNJ er)

n. A professionally dressed DEAFIE commuter who tells the driver he is deaf and therefore pays the handicapped fare instead of the normal fare.

SHORTHAND
(SHORT hand)

n. Any system of quick signing, such as SPLING.

SHORT-LEASHED

(SHORT leeshd)

adj. That disquieting feeling a hired interpreter often has after a few, long days of being reined in everywhere by a scurrying DEAFIE at a boring convention in some nice, scenic resort.

SHORT-ORDER DINER

(SHORT OR der DY ner)

n. A hungry DEAFIE who, even though he very much prefers cheeseburgers to hot dogs, orders one (1) hot dog, just because it is easier to pronounce.

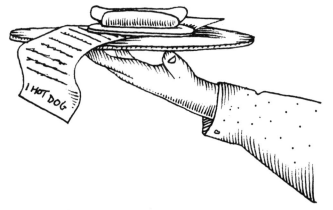

SHOW 'N' SIGN
(shoh en SYN)

v. What cute, young DEAFIE kids do when called up to the front of the class.

SIBBLING
(SIB ling)

n. Babbling in sign language by DEAFIE pre-schoolers.

SIGNATIVE
(SYN uh tive)

adj. A term that aptly describes a **VOSIGNFEROUS BIG HAND** who could not **KEEP HIS HANDS SHUT**.

SIGNATURE
(SIG nuh chur)

n. One's name in sign language.

SIGNIFICANT
(sig NIF i kuhnt)

adj. Magnificent in signing.

SIGNIFICANT FIGURES
(sig NIF i kuhnt FIG yuhrz)

n. Magnificent signers.

SIGNING TO THE WALL
(SYN ing to thuh wawl)

n. (A pathological behavior) Talking to the wall with one's hands.

SIGNONYM
(SYN oh nim)

n. One of two or more signs that have the same meaning.

SIGNOPAUSES
(SYN oh pawzuz)

n. Those little time lapses a lecturer builds into a technical dissertation so that the interpreter can catch up.

SIGNORA
(seen YOHR uh)

n. A married female who signs like an Italian.

SIGNOSIS
(sy NOH sis)

n. That hypnotic state, akin to sleeping, which can be induced by watching a boring signer. Often accompanied by IDIOT'S NOD.

SIGNS OF ZODIAC
(SYNZ of ZOHD ee ak)

n. Language used by DEAFIE astrologers.

SIGNTIFIC METHOD
(syn TIF ik METH uhd)

n. Procedure of observation and recording by **DEAFOLOGISTS**.

SIGNY
(SYN ee)

adj. Wordy.

SIMULIST
(SI muh list)

n. A hybrid between an oralist and a manualist.

SIMULIST'S AXIOM
(SI muh list es AKS see uhm)

n. The whole is greater than the sum of the ten supple fingers and one big mouth.

SIMULTIED-UP

(SI muhl tyd uhp)

adj. How an interpreter suddenly feels when he stops interpreting two agitated DEAFIES signing at the same time in a SIGNITION.

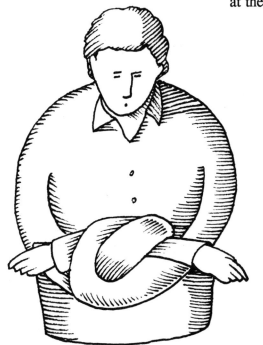

SKREWED UP
(SKREWD uhp)

adj. 1. That dreadful feeling a DEAFIE experiences when his TDD suddenly stops working during a **TYPEVERSATION**. 2. That same feeling also experienced by the guy at the other end of the line.

SK-SK-SK
(ES KAY ES KAY ES KAY)

v. (Telecommunications jargon) To overkill what appears to be a long-dead telephone line.

SLIGHT OF HAND
(slyt of HAND)

exp. Saying one thing, while signing something else completely different.

SLIP OF THE FINGER
(slip of thuh FING er)

n. (Same as **FREUDIAN SIGN.**)

SMIL^{EEEEEEEEEEEE}

(SMYL EEEEEEEEEEEE)

n. That distracting high-pitched sound emitted from a DEAFIE's hearing aid whenever he smiles.

SONIC BARRIER

(SON ik BAR ee er)

n. That invisible, mythical wall of HEARIE resistance to DEAFIES' advancement.

SONIC BOOM

(SON ik boom)

n. A shock wave produced by an explosive mixture of HEARCULEAN willpower and MYTHICIDE.

SOUNDING BOARD

(SOWN ding bord)

n. A HEARIE whom DEAFIES often sound out for his insight. (Compare with POUNDING BOARD.)

SOUNDPROOF

(SOWND proof)

adj. The reason why DEAFIES make excellent roommates for phone-hogging HEARIES.

SPECS-SPECKS

(SPEKS SPEKS)

n. 1. All these tiny, bothersome, SIGNFERENCING "spots" on the lens of a DEAFIE's eyeglasses. 2. (singular) EYESOGRE.

SPEED OF POUND

(speed of POUND)

n. Three times the speed of sound. (Applies only to **POUND WAVES.**)

STALLER

(STAWL er)

n. A DEAFIE found sitting in a bathroom stall during a fire alarm.

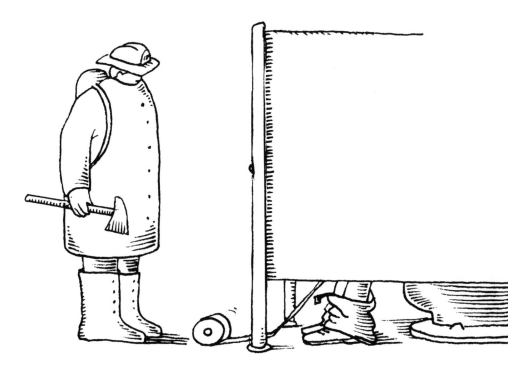

STAMPEDE
(stam PEED)

n. A herd of **ATTENSTOMPING** DEAFIES.

STARE FORCE
(STAYR FORS)

n. That hidden force of guilt that prevents a DEAFIE kid from daydreaming or looking elsewhere and keeps him riveted to his interpreter during a boring class lesson. (Compare with **PEER PRESSURE**.)

STARVEGAZERS
(starv gayz erz)

n. Those salivating DEAFIES standing at the food counter ogling at each tray to see if the order number matches theirs.

STOMPATTENED
(STOMP ah TEND)

adj. Being alerted to a **ATTENSTOMPER**'s calling.

STONE-HEARING
(STOHN HEER ing)

adj. (Same as **PROFOUNDLY HEARING**.)

STOP SIGN
(STOP syn)

n. That most annoying hand sign held right in front of a talking/signing DEAFIE by a HEARIE who suddenly answers his ringing phone.

STRAY-TUNED
(STRAY tewnd)

adj. Out of sync in communication, such as when an interpreter signs in ASL to an oral DEAFIE.

SUPERSONIC
(SOO pur SAWN ik)

adj. Too **PROFOUNDLY HEARING**.

SWIVELITIS
(SWIV uh LIT uhs)

n. That aching neck pain brought about from *not* standing on the recommended ELEVEQUILIBRIUM when waiting for an elevator.

SYN
(syn)

n. A pun in sign language, such as passing your eyes with the "milk" sign for "Pasteurized Milk."

"TAKE BOTH WAYS"
(tayk bohth wayz)

v. phr. (Author's family motto) 1. To look both ways before crossing the street. 2. To take care of oneself. (Often **LICENSE-PLATED** to "TBW" in **TYPEVERSATIONS**.)

TAKE SIGNS RIGHT OUT OF ONE'S HANDS
(tayk SYNZ RYT OWT of wunz handz)

v. phr. To sign what another was just about to sign.

TEEPHONE
(TEE fohn)

v. (Telecommunications jargon.) To type to by TDD < please ~ me, when you get home >.

THEORY OF RELATIVITY
(THEE uh ree of rel uh TIV uht ee)

n. A complicated theory that attempts to explain why so many relatives of a DEAFORMED DEAFIE are also deaf.

TOKENIZED
(toh KEN yzd)

adj. Being the only DEAFIE in a herd of babbling HEARIES (or vice versa with "flailing" instead of "babbling").

TOO MANY EYES HERE
(yoo MEN ee YZ heer)

exp. The reason why you should **KEEP YOUR HANDS SHUT**.

TYPEVERSATION

(TYP ver SAY shun)   n. A leisurely chat on TDD's.

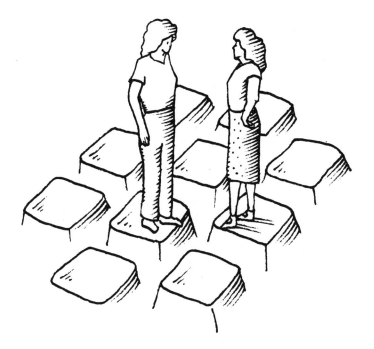

UNDEAF
(un DEF)

v. To try to convince a DEAFIE that it has *nothing* to do with his **INVISBLE HANDICAP**.

UNDERHAND
(uhn der HAND)

a. Lying with one's hands.

UNDERSHANDING
(uhn der SHAN ding)

n. 1. Comprehension of one's signing. 2. Interpretation of one's signing.

UNDESIGN
(uhn di SYN)

v. To make something more appealing to **ASLIANS**. (See **MANUAL TEST** for an example.)

UNGACIOUS
(uhn GAY shus)

adj. A term that best describes a **TYPEVERSATOR** who does not readily respond to an incoming "GA" and instead helps himself first to a leisurely cup of coffee.

UNSEESONED
(un SEEZ uhnd)

adj. Distastefully dark.

UNSIGNTLY
(un SYNT lee)

adj. (Sign language jargon) Not pleasing to the eye; ugly.

UNSOUNDING BOARD
(un SOWND ing bord)

n. A HEARIE whose head is so thick he appears to be "deaf."

UNSPILMANIZE

(un SPIL man yz)   v. To overthrow.

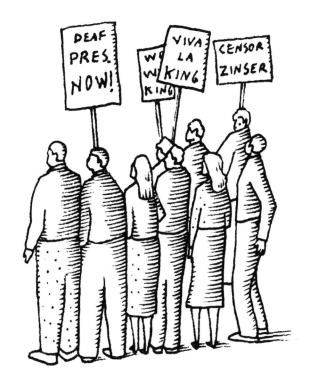

UNSTREAMED
(un STREEMD)

adj. Not mainstreamed or MINORSTREAMED.

UP IN ARMS
(UHP in armz)

adj. phr. Very agitated and **VOSIGNFEROUS** < DEAFIE students at Gallaudet University were ~ when they first **EYED** that Zinser was selected the new president >.

UP TO ONE'S EYES
(UHP too wuhnz YZ)

adv. phr. What **FACEDOWNERS** need to be reminded of again and again.

UPPLAUD
(uhp PLAWD)

v. To cheer on by waving with one's raised hands.

VACUUMIZED

(VAK yew uh myzd)

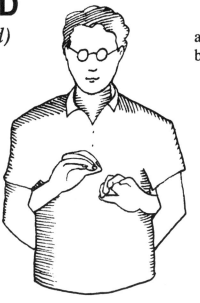

adj. How a DEAFIE feels once he realizes he has been VACSUCKERED.

VENTRILOSIGNING

(ven TRIL uh syn ing)

v. 1. Throwing one's hands into someone else's **ATMOSTPHERE**, such as by signing in front of him from behind. 2. Throwing one's signs into her/his dummy's gesturing hand.

VOCAL DISCORDS
(VOH kuhl DIS kordz)

n. (Medical term) The pair of folds of mucous membranes usually found in the Adam's Apple of manualists.

VOICEOVER
(VOYS oh ver)

n. That die-hard habit of oral DEAFIES who never turn off their vocal box even while talking with other DEAFIES.

VOSIGNFEROUS
(voh SYN fer uhs)

adj. Visually "loud."

WE THE PEOPLE
(WEE thuh PEE puhl)

n. phr. formal. DEAFIES, DEARIES, HEAFIES, and HEARIES - not necessarily in that order.

WHEELER-DEALER

(WEE ler DEE ler)

Any ignorant airport staffer who offers traveling DEAFIES a wheelchair unnecessarily.

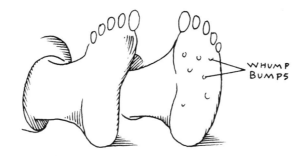

$$W_L - W_R = \Delta F$$

WHUMP BUMP

(WUHMP BUHMP)

n. One of those hardened blisters found only on the soles of **ATTENSTOMPING** DEAFIES' feet. (Note to all **DEAFOLOGISTS:** The difference in densities of **WHUMP BUMPS** on both feet is directly proportional to **DELTA FOOT**.)

WHYMEWHYMEWHYME

(WY mee WY mee WY mee)

adj. That feeling a **TOKENIZED** HEARIE in a group of DEAFIE diners always experiences when presented with a check by the waiter.

XOXOXO

(ksoh ksoh ksoh)

v. (Telecommunications jargon) To type farewell on TDD with kisses and smacks.

YANKY-HANKY

(YANGK ee HANGK ee)

n. A handkerchief used in VISUCLAPPING.

YAWING ONE'S CHIN

(yaw ing wunz chin)

v. phr. (origin: Aeronautical *Yaw* to turn about the vertical axis) To turn someone else's chin so as to establish a VISUALINE.

YELPANSION
(yel PAN shun)

n. That brief, temporary swelling of one's **ATMOSTPHERE** when excited or surprised.

ZINSERED
(ZIN surd)

adj. Censored by DEAFIES.

ZOOED
(ZOOD)

adj. The feeling a DEAFIE experiences when being pointed at by a HEARIE kid wondering out loud why he was talking funny.

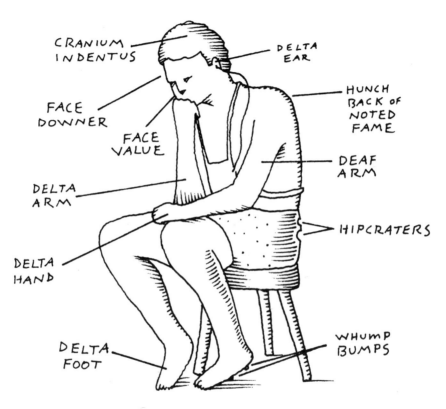

CRANIUM INDENTUS

DELTA EAR

HUNCH BACK OF NOTED FAME

FACE DOWNER

FACE VALUE

DEAF ARM

DELTA ARM

HIPCRATERS

DELTA HAND

DELTA FOOT

WHUMP BUMPS

THE THINKING DEAFIE

Official DEAFINITIONS Entry Form

(Make as many copies of this form as you wish.)

Dear Ken:

Here's a new **DEAFINITION** I've just invented. I understand that submission of this **DEAFINITION** constitutes my permission for it to be published in any future product and, if it is accepted, I will receive a free copy of the product.

SIGNLET: _____

DEAFINITION: _____
_____
_____

Sincerely, _____
(Signature)
Name: _____
Street: _____
City, State, Zip: _____

DiKen Products
9201 Long Branch Parkway
Silver Spring, Maryland 20901

Attention: Ken Glickman

Official DEAFINITIONS Entry Form

(Make as many copies of this form as you wish.)

Dear Ken:

Here's a new **DEAFINITION** I've just invented. I understand that submission of this **DEAFINITION** constitutes my permission for it to be published in any future product and, if it is accepted, I will receive a free copy of the product.

SIGNLET: _____

DEAFINITION: _____
_____
_____

Sincerely, _____
(Signature)

Name: _____
Street: _____
City, State, Zip: _____

DiKen Products
9201 Long Branch Parkway
Silver Spring, Maryland 20901

Attention: Ken Glickman

Official DEAFINITIONS Entry Form

(Make as many copies of this form as you wish.)

Dear Ken:

Here's a new **DEAFINITION** I've just invented. I understand that submission of this **DEAFINITION** constitutes my permission for it to be published in any future product and, if it is accepted, I will receive a free copy of the product.

SIGNLET: _____

DEAFINITION: _____
_____
_____

Sincerely, _____
(Signature)
Name: _____
Street: _____
City, State, Zip: _____

DiKen Products
9201 Long Branch Parkway
Silver Spring, Maryland 20901

Attention: Ken Glickman